# GET HOLD: UNCONTROLLABLE BOWEL SYNDROME (IBS)

**Dr. Philip G. Rhode**

# TABLE OF CONTENT

# Chapter 1

IBS and It's Symptoms:

You might have just heard the term "IBS" and been curious about what it means. To put it another way, it is a medical condition in which the bowel is unable to effectively perform its normal functions, despite its simplicity. Additionally, that condition is known as Irritable Bowel Syndrome (IBS). Irritable bowel syndrome, or IBS, is characterized by unpleasant or painful abdominal symptoms. Common IBS symptoms include gas, bloating, constipation, and diarrhea. IBS doesn't harm your gastrointestinal system or raise your gamble for colon malignant growth. Changing your diet and way of life can often help you manage your symptoms. Irritable bowel syndrome, or IBS, is a group of digestive system-related symptoms. It is a common but unpleasant gastrointestinal condition. IBS is a type of functional gastrointestinal (GI) disorder in which individuals experience excessive gas, abdominal pain, and cramps. These conditions, which are also known as disorders of gut-brain interaction, are caused by issues with how your gut and brain interact. Your digestive system becomes extremely sensitive as a result of these issues. Additionally, they alter the way your bowel muscles contract. Constipation, diarrhea, and pain in the stomach are the consequences.

Different types of Irritable Bowel Syndrome (IBS):
IBS is categorized by researchers according to the kind of issues you have with your bowel movements. This sort of IBS can influence your treatment. Certain medications are only effective for specific types of IBS. People with IBS frequently experience abnormal bowel movements on some days and normal bowel movements on others.

The type of IBS you have depends on the abnormal bowel movements you experience: Constipation-related Irritable Bowel Syndrome (IBS-C): The majority of your poop is lumpy and hard.

Diarrheal Irritable Bowel Syndrome (IBS-D): The majority of your poop is watery and loose.

Irritable bowel syndrome (IBS) is characterized by irregular bowel movements (IBS-M): On the same day, you experience loose, watery bowel movements in addition to hard, lumpy bowel movements.

Only a small percentage of IBS sufferers experience severe symptoms. Diet, lifestyle, and stress management can sometimes be used to control symptoms in some people. Medication and counseling can be used to treat symptoms that are more severe. The colon muscle tends to contract more in people with IBS than in people without the condition. Cramps and pain are caused by these contractions. Additionally, people with IBS typically have lower pain tolerance. IBS sufferers may also have an excess of bacteria in their gastrointestinal (GI) tract, which may contribute to their symptoms, according to research.

Other names for Irritable Bowel Syndrome (IBS) You may hear these names for IBS: **Irritable bowel, Irritable colon and Spastic colon.**

Symptoms of Irritable Bowel syndrome: stomach, as symptoms frequently occur when you are experiencing emotional stress, tension, and anxiety. If you experience other IBS symptoms or persistent changes in your bowel habits, see a doctor. They might be a sign of something more serious, like colon cancer. Among the more serious symptoms are: Anemia caused by iron deficiency, nighttime diarrhea, rectal bleeding, weight loss, unexplained vomiting, pain that doesn't go away with gas or a bowel movement, etc.

IBS has a variety of symptoms, but they typically last for a long time. The most typical are: Symptoms associated with passing a bowel movement include abdominal pain, cramping, or bloating; changes in the appearance of a bowel movement; changes in the frequency with which you have a bowel movement; and the sensation of an incomplete evacuation and an increase in gas or mucus in the stool.

In addition, IBS is associated with:
Poor quality of life: The quality of life for many people with moderate to severe IBS is poor. According to research, people who have IBS miss three times as many days of work as people who don't have bowel symptoms.

Mood disorders: Having IBS symptoms can make you feel depressed or anxious. Discouragement and nervousness additionally can exacerbate IBS. IBS can occasionally cause symptoms for many people. However, the syndrome is more likely to affect you;

If you are young; IBS is more common in younger people under the age of 50.

If you are a woman; Women are more likely than men to experience IBS in the United States. IBS is also a risk factor when women take estrogen therapy before or after menopause.

If you Have a family history of IBS: Genes, shared factors in a family, or a combination of genes and environment may all play a role. suffer from depression, anxiety, or other mental health issues. A history of emotional, sexual, or physical abuse may also be a risk factor.

Bloating, abdominal pain, and discomfort are all symptoms of IBS, also known as irritable bowel syndrome. Even though this disorder does not pose a threat to one's life, its symptoms can make living with them very difficult and painful. The following is a list of a few issues that can arise from this condition.

Additional Symptoms:

Although stomach pain, diarrhea, and constipation are the most common symptoms of IBS, other symptoms can also occur. Although the following may appear unrelated to IBS upon initial examination, they provide your healthcare provider with a more comprehensive picture.

As a result, it's critical to keep track of and discuss all of your symptoms with your doctor. Other areas of the body that hurt: problems sleeping, heart palpitations, dizziness, bladder urgency, increased frequency of the need to urinate, fatigue, pain during menstruation, pain during sexual activity, and other symptoms.

# Chapter 2

Triggers and Complications of Irritable Bowel Syndrome:
You can devise a strategy to avoid the triggers that can aggravate your IBS symptoms once you are aware of them. You will be able to work on reducing the number of issues you have with bloating, constipation, diarrhea, and stomach pain as a result.
IBS is different for everybody, except it might assist with monitoring how you respond to the most widely recognized side effects and figuring out how to forestall them.

The exact cause of IBS isn't known. Factors that appear to play a role include:
Muscle contractions in the intestine; Layers of muscle line the walls of the intestines, which contract as food moves through your digestive tract. Gas, bloating, and diarrhea can result from more intense and prolonged

contractures. Food passage may be slowed by weak contractions, resulting in hard, dry stools.

Nervous system; When your stomach stretches from gas or stool, discomfort may be caused by digestive system nerve issues. Inadequately organized signals between the mind and the digestion tracts can make your body blow up to changes that commonly happen in the stomach-related process. This can cause diarrhea, pain, or constipation.

Severe infection; After a severe bout of diarrhea brought on by a virus or bacteria, IBS can occur. Gastroenteritis is the name for this. Overgrowth of bacteria in the intestines (IBS) may also be associated with it.

Early life stress; IBS symptoms typically appear more frequently in people who have been exposed to stressful situations, particularly as children.

Changes in gut microbes; Changes in bacteria, fungi, and viruses, which typically live in the intestines and are important to health, are one example. According to research, the microbes of IBS sufferers may differ from those of non-IBS sufferers. Hemorrhoids can result from persistent diarrhea or constipation.

1. Diet Triggers for IBS Constipation:
The following foods can exacerbate constipation caused by IBS: Refined grains in cereals and bread, processed foods like chips and cookies, coffee, carbonated beverages, and alcohol, high-protein diets, and dairy products like cheese

Better Diet Choices for Constipation:
Increase your daily fiber intake by 2 to 3 grams until you reach 25 grams for women or 38 grams for men. Whole-grain bread, cereals, beans, fruits, and vegetables are all good sources. Consume dried plums and

prune juice, which are high in the sugar substitute sorbitol, in moderation. Every day, sip a lot of plain water. Try flaxseed ground up. Sprinkle it on cooked vegetables and salads.

2. Diet Triggers for IBS Diarrhea:
Food sources that can aggravate IBS for certain individuals include Too much fiber, especially the insoluble kind found in fruits and vegetable skins; foods and beverages containing chocolate, alcohol, caffeine, fructose, or sorbitol; large meals; fried and fatty foods; dairy products, particularly for individuals who are unable to digest lactose in dairy products a condition known as lactose intolerance; and foods containing wheat for individuals who are allergic to or have a negative reaction to gluten.

Better Diet Choices for Diarrhea:
Consuming a small amount of soluble fiber can bulk up your stools. Whole-wheat bread, oats, barley, brown rice, whole-grain pasta,

fruit flesh (not skin), and dried fruits are all good sources. Consuming ice-cold water and steaming hot soup during the same meal is not recommended. Avoid eating cabbage, onions, and broccoli. They can make you feel worse by releasing gas. If you think you might have a wheat allergy, talk to your doctor or a dietitian. Drink water an hour before or after meals, not while you eat. Try to stay away from foods that make you feel gas and bloated, like beans, Brussels sprouts, wheat germ, raisins, and celery.

3. Stress and Anxiety Triggers for IBS:
Anxiety and stress can exacerbate IBS symptoms. There are many different causes of anxiety, including Work, your commute, home issues, financial issues, and the feeling that you can't control everything

How to Manage Stress:
Make healthy choices. Eat a diet that works for your IBS that is well-balanced. Get enough sleep and regular exercise, as well as

as much fun as you can. Take a walk, read, listen to music, or read. With behavioral therapy, you can learn better ways to calm down. There are several kinds: psychotherapy, biofeedback, hypnosis, relaxation therapy, and cognitive behavioral therapy. Talk about your IBS with your family, close friends, boss, or coworkers if you feel comfortable doing so. They are better able to support you and comprehend how it affects you when they know what's going on.

4. Drugs That Can Trigger IBS:
Constipation and diarrhea can be brought on by some drugs. IBS sufferers may struggle with Some antidepressants, antibiotics, and sorbitol-based medications like cough syrup.

How to Choose Better Meds:
Consider switching to a medication that won't worsen your symptoms with your doctor. But before you stop taking your

medication, ask them. Choose your antidepressants carefully. Tricyclic antidepressants, which are older medications, can cause constipation. Standard ones, such as fluoxetine (Prozac, Sarafem) and sertraline (Zoloft), which are known as selective serotonin reuptake inhibitors, can cause diarrhea. Find the best one by working with your doctor.

5. Menstrual Triggers for IBS:
During their periods, women with IBS typically experience worse symptoms. You can alleviate pain and discomfort during that time of the month, but you cannot prevent it.

How to Feel Better:
Consider purchasing contraceptives. They might help you get your periods more often. However, they may result in side effects such as diarrhea, constipation, vomiting, stomach cramps, or bloating. Find one that

works without causing additional problems by working with your doctor.

Deal with severe PMS. Ask your doctor for advice on which depression medications might be beneficial.

6. Other Triggers:
Eating too quickly, chewing gum, not getting enough exercise, and eating while driving or working.

What to Do:
Avoid being distracted while you eat. Attempt to exercise for at least 30 minutes each day. It can ease stress and prevent constipation. Also, discuss all of your treatment options for IBS with diarrhea and IBS with constipation with your doctor.

Complications to Lifestyle:
The prevalence of irritable bowel syndrome (IBS) among Canadians is one of the highest in the world. As a result, IBS is a leading cause of workplace absenteeism in Canada,

which is not surprising. What's more, since it's normally a long-lasting condition, people with IBS frequently need clinical help across their life expectancy. It can cause a number of issues if it is not treated.

However, IBS symptoms can make it difficult to get medical care. It can be challenging to travel to an appointment due to unpredictable diarrhea as well as gas and bloating that is unpleasant. In addition, many Canadians either lack a family doctor or cannot obtain timely medical care. As a result, their quality of life can be severely impacted as they struggle alone with severe IBS symptoms. In more ways than one, IBS is somewhat mysterious. Not only is its underlying cause unknown, but neither can it be tested for. Because of this, determining whether you have IBS or something else can be challenging. Because of this, IBS is a diagnosis of exclusion, which means that your doctor will only diagnose it if all other possibilities have been ruled out.

Doctors believe that IBS is partly caused by your brain being overly sensitive to the sensation of food passing through your digestive tract, although the exact cause is unknown. This theory has been supported by studies of neuroimaging, which have shown that parts of the brain that control attention, emotion, and pain have changed. Consequently, it is referred to as a disorder of gut-brain interaction or a functional gastrointestinal disorder. The immune system and the permeability of the digestive tract's mucosal lining may also be factors in IBS. Hormones may also play a role because it is more common in women.

Signs and symptoms of severe Irritable Bowel Syndrome (IBS):
IBS can be very bad, and many people say that their symptoms make their quality of life worse.
Some examples include:
Constipation that causes straining, which can result in hemorrhoids, diarrhea, and

fecal urgency, which can result in incontinence due to their unpredictability, stool volume, and consistency, feeling like you haven't emptied your bowels completely, low energy and fatigue due to both connectivities within a network in the brain and immune activation are all symptoms of IBS.

Irritable Bowel syndrome (IBS) risk factors:
It is unclear why some people develop IBS while others do not. It is possible to have the condition but not have any risk factors, or to have many risk factors but not develop IBS. Nevertheless, you are more likely to receive an IBS diagnosis if:
You an ongoing smoker, Are between your youngsters and your 40s, Have somebody in your family with IBS, You Are a lady, Were presented to injury, for example, adolescence misuse, Had a gastric occasion, for example, a parasite disease or food contamination, Consistently experience high feelings of anxiety, Have mental

comorbidity, somewhere close to 50-90% of patients with IBS likewise have a dysfunctional behavior, particularly summed up nervousness confusion and gloom. While the causes of symptom flare-ups are better understood, the causes of IBS are still unknown. It's a good idea to write down your specific triggers in a journal, but here are some more general ones:

Alcohol;
Alcohol makes digestion go faster and is hard on the stomach. This can significantly aggravate symptoms, particularly diarrhea.

Certain foods:
There are no specific foods that cause IBS, despite the fact that each person will likely have their own specific dietary no-go areas. However, a lot of people have issues with caffeine, fried foods, and some artificial sweeteners. Eating late at night and frequently skipping meals can also be

problematic. Keep a food journal and talk to a dietitian if you're not sure about your trigger foods and want to make sure you're eating a well-balanced diet without them.

Some medications:
IBS flare-ups are frequently brought on by antibiotics, which alter the flora of your intestinal tract. In contrast, antidepressants can both exacerbate IBS symptoms and cause flare-ups. Sadly, determining whether an antidepressant will exacerbate or alleviate your condition may require trial and error based on your doctor's prescription. Before taking any medication, I always recommend consulting your doctor.

Stress:
Your digestive system and your brain communicate in both directions through the gut-brain axis. Even though this is a vital information pathway for your body, it also means that stress frequently causes IBS symptoms.

How to know if IBS is severe;
Your doctor cannot assess the severity of your IBS symptoms because the inside of your colon appears normal. In the end, it all depends on how much it is affecting your life. Your condition is severe if you are unable to effectively manage your IBS symptoms so that you can work, study, sleep, or socialize.

How to treat severe IBS;
IBS has no treatment. Therefore, the goal of treatment for severe IBS is to reduce and control symptoms. Since both exercise and dietary changes have been shown to lessen symptoms, this should include both.
Whether you're experiencing diarrhea, constipation, or a combination of the two, adding fiber to your diet can be beneficial because it helps to absorb water and bulk up your stool. Eating more fruits and vegetables or taking a powder or pill with fiber can help. But be aware that increasing your fiber intake without increasing your

water intake will result in the opposite, so if you decide to do this, make sure to drink more water. All of these interventions, on the other hand, take time to work, making them good long-term solutions but not very helpful during an acute attack. So, in cases of severe IBS pain, what should you do? According to research, peppermint oil can successfully alleviate bloating and pain.

Additionally, many swear by heat. They say that warming up their stomachs with a heating pad or hot water bottle helps them feel better. Another way to get rid of cramping is to take diarrheal medications that are sold over the counter. It is best to consult a doctor to rule out the possibility of another medical condition if severe IBS symptoms have become the norm, symptoms onset after age 50, rectal bleeding, nocturnal diarrhea, unexplained weight loss, or progressive abdominal pain are present. This is true regardless of the management strategies you use. They should also know if you have colorectal cancer or inflammatory bowel disease in your family.

They are able to give you prescriptions to help ease stomach pain and cramping if you need them. Alternatively, they might suggest taking antidepressants in smaller amounts, which can help stop the pain. Alternative treatments for IBS, such as prescription digital therapeutics like cognitive behavioral therapy (CBT), have also been approved by Health Canada.

Complications of IBS during pregnancy;
Although they aren't life-threatening, IBS complications can make your pregnancy more difficult. IBS, for instance, is linked to an increased risk of preeclampsia and deep vein thrombosis (a blood clot in a vein) during pregnancy, according to data. Additionally, it may raise the possibility of congenital birth defects in the baby as well as the risk of miscarriage and ectopic pregnancy. In addition, hormonal changes

brought on by pregnancy can exacerbate IBS symptoms. Additionally, pregnancy food cravings can cause you to consume foods that can aggravate your IBS. Additionally, attempting to alleviate symptoms through diet could deprive you and your baby of essential nutrients. As a result, getting in touch with a dietitian is a great way to make sure you and your child are eating well.

What happens if IBS is left untreated?
The answer to your question about whether untreated IBS can increase your risk of colon cancer is no. Your overall life expectancy will not be affected by IBS, nor will it progress into another digestive disorder. However, IBS can impair the quality of life. As a result, both mental and physical health issues can result from untreated IBS.
Some of the most common are these:

Hemorrhoids: Hemorrhoids are frequently a recurring problem with IBS and are brought on by the increased pressure that results from straining during a bowel movement. Although hemorrhoids can be treated, unless the underlying constipation is addressed, they are likely to recur.

Severe cramping and pain: IBS is characterized by severe stomach pain and cramping. The severity of the symptoms can make it difficult to sleep, work, or even leave the house in severe cases.

Bowel incontinence: At least once per month, nearly one in five people with IBS experience bowel incontinence. This can cause significant distress, which can have an effect on your mental health and your ability to work.

Pelvic floor dysfunction: Frequent constipation can strain your pelvic muscles, prompting pelvic floor brokenness. This can exacerbate existing constipation, lead to back pain, and cause urgency and incontinence in the urinate. When one or more of the organs in your pelvis, like your uterus, bladder, or bowel, move down into the vagina in women, this can occasionally result in pelvic floor prolapse.

Inadequate nutrition: By controlling their diet, many people with IBS experience relief from their symptoms. But if you stick to a strict diet like the low-FODMAP diet and don't replace bad foods with healthy ones, you might not get enough nutrients.

Mental health issues: There is ample evidence to support the existence of severe IBS-related mental health issues. The symptoms can be hard to predict, making it hard to go to the bathroom and restricting your behavior. This can make it difficult to socialize, study, or work, which can lead to mental health issues like depression and anxiety.

When to see a doctor for your IBS:

When your IBS symptoms change or get worse, you should talk to a doctor. Although IBS does not increase your risk of colorectal cancer, chronic diarrhea, constipation, gas, and bloating that are common to both conditions make it possible to miss the first signs of colon cancer if you have IBS. In a similar vein, you should immediately see a doctor if you have bleeding from your rectal area, blood in your stool, or unexplained weight loss. These aren't the usual side effects of an IBS flare-up and could point to other health issues.

Even if your symptoms have not changed, you should see a doctor if they are preventing you from doing things or making it hard for you to manage them.

You can get the help you need without having to leave the comfort of your own home by visiting an online doctor. In addition, if you require a prescription, they can issue one during your appointment and deliver it to your doorstep or to the pharmacy of your choice.

Alternatively, speaking with an online dietitian is a good idea if you want comprehensive dietary support for your IBS. While still ensuring that your body receives the vitamins, minerals, and calories it requires to remain healthy, a dietitian can assist you in controlling your symptoms. Furthermore, you don't have to miss work or fight the traffic to do so.

In the event that you feel like you're not in charge of your IBS, now is the right time to roll out an improvement. Symptoms can be managed with help. Contact a doctor right away to stop IBS from controlling your life.

IBS can result in physical issues that can have an impact on your way of life. You will be able to make the most of your circumstances as long as you are aware of them.

The four most typical and significant issues are outlined in the following bullet points:

Gastrointestinal Tract (GI) Disorders: Inflammation of the gastrointestinal tract, which includes the route that food travels from the mouth to the anus, is a hallmark of GI disorders. You might be given some tablets to treat mild cases, and in more severe cases, you might need surgery to fix the damaged tissue.

Diarrhea: When you have three or more liquid bowel movements per day, you have diarrhea. Antibiotics can be used to treat acute diarrhea, but in less severe cases, your doctor may prescribe products similar to Pepto-Bismol.

Cramping: Consuming an excessive amount of food is usually the cause of cramping. By reducing the amount of food consumed or by eating meals in smaller portions, cramping and diarrhea can be avoided. When used in conjunction with the solutions that are provided in this article, a healthy diet that is supervised by a dietitian can be beneficial.

Sleeping disturbances: Due to the fact that abdominal pain and other cramps may keep you awake at night, sleep issues are common with IBS. As a result, you'll have less energy throughout the day and feel more tired. A doctor might give you sleeping pills so that your body can rest if this problem gets too bad.

Complications of Depression and Anxiety:
It has been determined that three out of every four people with IBS will experience depression at some point. Depression encompasses more than just sadness. Extreme sadness, a loss of interest in hobbies and friends, drastic changes in eating habits, fatigue and insomnia, and even suicidal ideation are all symptoms of depression. To treat this entanglement, you might have to begin taking antidepressants,

which are drugs that assist with treating discouragement and its side effects.
Anxiety is another problem that IBS causes.

GAD, or generalized anxiety disorder, strikes about half of all IBS patients. People with this chronic condition experience extreme anxiety and unease regarding a wide range of issues and circumstances. CBT, or cognitive behavioral therapy, is one treatment for anxiety.
By attempting to alter a patient's thinking and behavior, this talking therapy assists the patient in coping with current issues. In order to determine what causes your anxiety, each problem is broken down into smaller components. By avoiding these negative triggers and concentrating on the more positive aspects of life, patients can better manage their anxiety in this manner.

Other Physical Complications:
Constipation and issues with the bladder are two additional IBS complications. You

might feel like you're constipated or have hard-to-pass bowel movements or infrequent ones. Bladder issues might turn into an issue too, for tension in the bladder might cause sporadic pee and bother. In addition, IBS may cause muscle pain and heartburn in your body.

Your normal way of life may also be put in jeopardy by IBS complications. Due to the difficulty, you may have to cope with your symptoms outside of the home and in relationships, you may have difficulty leaving the house and enjoying a healthy sexual life. However, don't allow your IBS to make you pull out from a charming life.

# Chapter 3

Treatment Options and How to Manage Irritable Bowel Syndrome (IBS):
Your doctor may suggest a number of tests, including stool tests, to see if there is an infection. Stool studies can also determine whether your intestines are having trouble absorbing nutrients. Malabsorption is the name of this condition. In order to rule out other causes of your symptoms, additional tests may be suggested.

Diagnostic procedures can include:
Colonoscopy: Your provider examines the entire length of the colon with a small, flexible tube.

CT scan: If you have belly pain, this test may rule out other possible causes of your symptoms by producing images of your pelvis and abdomen.

Upper endoscopy: The esophagus, which is the tube that connects your mouth and stomach, is reached by inserting a long, flexible tube down your throat. Your healthcare provider will be able to see your upper digestive tract thanks to a camera on the tube's end. A biopsy, or tissue sample, may be taken during an endoscopy. In order to check for bacterial overgrowth, a fluid sample may be taken. If celiac disease is suspected, an endoscopy may be suggested.

Laboratory tests can include Tests for lactose intolerance: You need an enzyme called lactase to break down the sugar in dairy products. If you don't make lactase, you might have symptoms like gas, diarrhea, and stomach pain that are similar to IBS. Your doctor might order a breath test or tell you to stop eating milk and milk products for a few weeks.

Breath test for bacterial overgrowth: A breath test can also tell you if your small intestine has too many bacteria. People who have had bowel surgery, diabetes, or another disease that slows digestion are more likely to have bacterial overgrowth.

Stool tests: It's possible that bacteria, parasites, or bile acid will be found in your stool. Your liver makes bile acid, a digestive fluid.

The goal of IBS treatment is to alleviate symptoms so that you can live as pain-free a life as possible. Changing your diet and lifestyle, as well as managing your stress, are often effective ways to control mild symptoms. Try to: Eat foods high in fiber, drink a lot of fluids, exercise frequently, and get enough sleep to manage your symptoms.

Your provider might suggest that you eliminate from your diet:
1. High-gas foods; Avoid carbonated and alcoholic beverages as well as certain foods

that may make you feel gassier if you have bloating or gas.

2. Gluten; Even if they don't have celiac disease, some people with IBS report feeling better when they stop eating gluten (wheat, barley, and rye).

3. FODMAPs; FODMAPs carbohydrates like lactose, fructose, and others may cause sensitivity in some individuals; polyols, oligosaccharides, disaccharides, and monosaccharides can be fermented. Certain grains, fruits, vegetables, and dairy products contain FODMAPs. The best natural treatment for IBS is thought to be a diet low in FODMAPs. Avoid these foods that are high in FODMAPs: Scallions, Soybeans, Cherries, Feijoa, Cranberry, Blackcurrant, Figs, Guava, Peaches, Watermelon, Mango, Honey, Malt syrup, Saccharin, and other vegetables are among the pickled items.

Instead, fill your diet with low-FODMAP foods that are less likely to trigger IBS.

Common low-FODMAP foods include: Bean sprouts, chives, broccoli, kale, carrots, cucumber, eggplant, zucchini, unripe bananas, fennel, pumpkin, spinach, turnip, spring onions, dragon fruit, orange, papaya, strawberry, raspberry, feta cheese, dark chocolate, and other similar items are among the options.

Many of those fruits and vegetables will be included in a low FODMAP diet, but remember that quantity is important. If you consume an excessive amount of food with fewer FODMAPs, you may experience symptoms.

Now you may be asking What are the benefits of an IBS diet?

The IBS diet helps treat a variety of gastrointestinal symptoms, such as abdominal distension, constipation, diarrhea, and pain.

1. All IBS subtypes (IBS-C, IBS-D, and IBS-M) benefited greatly from the low FODMAP diet, according to a 2021 study. The low-FODMAP diet has been shown to be an effective treatment for alleviating abdominal symptoms. Other studies backup these findings. Patients with IBS, particularly those with IBS-D, experienced significant reductions in their primary symptoms and increased stool output when they followed a diet low in FODMAPs. According to the findings of a large study that was published in 2016, people who eat a diet low in FODMAPs have a higher chance of experiencing less bloating and pain in the stomach by 81% and 75%, respectively.

2. Try intermittent fasting: A well-liked way to eat is intermittent fasting, which consists of timed periods of fasting. It involves restricting calories for 14 to 20 hours at a time, up to several days a week (or every day).

In humans, calorie restriction improves insulin sensitivity and blood pressure.

IBS treatment may include intermittent fasting. One clinical investigation discovered that fasting people had huge enhancements in 7 out of 8 IBS side effects, including IBS symptoms such as abdominal pain, abdominal distention, diarrhea, decreased appetite, nausea, anxiety, and quality of life, among other things, will affect how effective intermittent fasting is. Discuss with your doctor which method of fasting is best for you.

3. Exercise: Strength and cardiovascular fitness are improved through regular physical activity, resulting in improved health and longevity. One study found that IBS symptoms can be alleviated by engaging in low-intensity exercise.

According to a 2011 study, patients with IBS who are physically active have less severe symptoms than patients who are not physically active. Yoga is one of the best physical activities for IBS. Yoga is an exercise for the mind and body, and many of its postures are bodyweight training exercises that use your own weight as resistance. One hour of yoga consistently for quite a long time essentially further develops IBS side effects, as per a 2018 precise survey of accessible proof.

4. Reduce stress in your life: The hormone cortisol rises in response to chronic stress, which can have an effect on our digestion. As a result, controlling your stress and anxiety is crucial to controlling your IBS symptoms. Because IBS is a disorder that responds to stress, treating it must focus on controlling stress and the responses that stress causes. Up to 30% of people with IBS experience abdominal pain and distension as a result of stressful life events. Stress caused by IBS can be reduced in a variety of ways.

Try mindfulness meditation, for instance, which has been shown to be the best predictor of improvement in quality of life and gastrointestinal symptoms. As I mentioned earlier, yoga is also a great exercise for dealing with stress. In grown-ups with significant sadness, an 8-week yoga meditation brought about measurably huge decreases in sorrow seriousness. You can get rid of IBS and get back to living your life by practicing relaxation techniques and living a low-stress lifestyle.

5. Try biofeedback: Biofeedback is a mind-body treatment for IBS that is part of complementary and alternative medicine (CAM). Retraining the body to control specific responses is involved. Individuals are connected to sensors during biofeedback, which assist in monitoring physiological processes such as Breathing, Pulse, Skin sensations, Muscle withdrawals, and Temperature. Biofeedback has been

shown to reduce pain, reduce mental distress, and alleviate IBS symptoms in a number of small studies. People with IBS can intervene before their nervous system has a chance to negatively affect their GI function by using biofeedback to detect symptoms early. Biofeedback therapy has been shown to improve symptoms, such as more regular bowel movements, in 55% to 82% of patients over time, according to long-term studies.

A dietitian can help you with these diet changes. Counseling might be suggested by your doctor if your problems are moderate or severe, especially if you have depression or if stress tends to make your symptoms worse.

Based on your symptoms, medications may be recommended, including:
Anti-diarrheal medications, laxatives, and fiber supplements; When it comes to over-the-counter medications, anticholinergics, tricyclic antidepressants,

SSRI antidepressants, pain relievers, and so on, you should always seek advice from your physician.

So, if you always feel like you have a knot in your stomach, try one of these popular IBS remedies;

Probiotics;

Probiotics may be the natural treatment for irritable bowel syndrome that people love the most and use the most. IBS may be brought on by an imbalance between good and bad bacteria in the digestive tract in some instances. Good probiotic bacteria can help the gut properly digest food, prevent the growth of toxin-producing bacteria, and improve the balance of the intestinal flora. All of this helps alleviate the IBS symptoms of constipation, diarrhea, gas, bloating, and cramps. Yogurt and cheese are the best natural sources of probiotics; however, a probiotic supplement is frequently the choice of those who are lactose intolerant. You can tell a probiotic product's strength and effectiveness by looking for active live cultures when you buy one. When probiotics are added to a supplement, they are frequently paired with a prebiotic fiber like FOS, which helps probiotics grow once they reach the digestive tract.

Calcium;

Try a calcium supplement if you have IBS-D and diarrhea is your main concern. Better-formed stools are made possible by this essential mineral's ability to reduce the amount of water in the intestines and encourage the contraction of the gut muscles. Dairy products contain a lot of lactose and fat, both of which can exacerbate IBS symptoms, so IBS diets often lack calcium. White beans, sardines, and kale are examples of dairy-free calcium sources that can be beneficial. The majority of calcium supplements are a convenient alternative and do not contain lactose.

Calcium carbonate, which can be taken three times a day in doses of up to 500 milligrams, is the type of calcium supplement that works best to treat diarrhea. If you have mostly constipation-type IBS, calcium should be avoided in high doses and replaced with a magnesium supplement.

Fiber;
In addition to stabilizing intestinal contractions and restoring normal bowel function, fiber absorbs water from the intestines to firm and bulk up stools, making them easier to pass. But for some people with IBS, fiber can be a double-edged sword, so it's important to think about the kind of fiber you're eating.
Rice, pasta, oatmeal, beets, bananas, mangoes, and potatoes all contain soluble fiber, which should serve as the foundation for all meals and snacks and is frequently well tolerated. In contrast, there is a wide range of tolerance for foods with insoluble fiber, such as whole grains, cereals, bran, nuts, and seeds. Consumption of these foods

may need to be restricted. One of the best sources of soluble fiber is psyllium husks. It is especially beneficial for IBS sufferers who fluctuate between constipation and diarrhea when taken as a supplement because it both loosens and thickens stools. In order to avoid gas and bloating, gradually increase your fiber intake to approximately 30 grams per day and drink plenty of water. Due to the way they are broken down in the intestines, fiber supplements typically cause less gas and bloating than dietary fiber.

Peppermint Oil;
One of the strongest herbs for relieving spasmodic pain, peppermint is especially helpful for people who suffer from gas and bloating. The oil has menthol in it, which helps relax and calm the stomach and intestinal muscles, easing spasms. 75% of the people in a recent study who took peppermint oil capsules daily for four weeks reported significantly lessening symptoms of IBS. Take peppermint as a digestive aid

after eating a lot or when cramps and bloating occur. For long-term relief, simply infuse peppermint leaves in hot water or take peppermint supplements.

Ginger;
Strong digestive enzymes found in ginger root alleviate diarrhea-related nausea and cramps in the intestines. Additionally, the herb has mild anti-inflammatory properties that alleviate abdominal discomfort and pain. It's not difficult to add new ginger root to your feasts and solidified ginger can likewise make a helpful tidbit. Alternatively, you can make your own ginger tea by grating the root into hot water, straining, and sweetening it with honey. For long-term relief, ginger supplements can be taken daily and are best taken with food.

Additional Tips for Living With IBS:
Fortunately, many individuals with IBS are able to successfully manage their symptoms by altering their diet and lifestyle. Attempt a

sensitivity-end diet by cutting normal triggers like dairy, wheat, citrus, and sweet food varieties. After that, gradually include foods again in your diet.

Distress. Stress is a common cause of IBS symptoms, so de-stress and unwind every day. Yoga and meditation should be your primary focus.

Visit your doctor if you think you are experiencing symptoms of IBS to rule out other possible causes and receive a diagnosis. They will also assist you in creating a treatment plan and finding IBS treatments that meet your specific requirements.

Home remedies for Irritable Bowel Syndrome: IBS (irritable bowel syndrome) can be greatly managed with the assistance of natural treatments. On the other hand, it's always best to choose a treatment that works best for your body. IBS affects approximately 11% of the global population, making it an increasingly common condition. IBS management and the options for treating IBS.

Our gut is extremely sensitive to stress and inflammatory foods, as previously mentioned. The expert suggests limiting your intake of inflammatory foods and focusing on cooling foods like melons and astringent fruits like apples, berries, and cherries instead. The expert has recommended the best ways to alleviate your symptoms and feel better.

Here are some products that you can try:
1. Count on soaked coriander or sabja seeds
The expert suggests soaking one teaspoon of coriander seeds overnight and drinking the water on an empty stomach the next morning. Because they cool your intestines, you can even chew on the seeds.
Alternatively, you could soak one teaspoon of sabja or sweet basil seeds overnight in water in a bowl or bottle. They swell and have an outer layer that looks like gel. Drink this throughout the day or on an empty

stomach in the morning. It reduces inflammation while also cooling your gut.

2. Add astringent foods to your diet
Pomegranates and bananas are two fruits that help keep diarrhea-like symptoms at bay and help keep the stools together. For those who are experiencing these symptoms, the only two fruits that should be consumed immediately following a meal are these two. Otherwise, the expert advises keeping an hour's gap between meals and fruits.

3. Coconut water can be a healthy remedy
You can drink a lot of tender coconut water made from fresh coconut meat, which also cools your intestines. You must also get in touch with a doctor right away to use herbs and medications to get rid of these symptoms.

4. Aloe Vera
You Will Need
2-4 ounces of aloe vera juice

What You Need To Do
Polish off 2-4 ounces of aloe vera squeeze once every day. Before trying this, talk to your doctor to make sure it won't affect any of your other medications.

How Often You Should Do This
You can drink this once daily or as prescribed by your physician.
Why This Works: Consuming juice made from aloe vera can help alleviate IBS symptoms. These advantages may be due to its laxative and anti-inflammatory properties. However, this treatment is only suitable for short-term use.

The bottom line
IBS can be painful and difficult to treat. However, you can take preventative measures to lessen symptoms and improve gut function. You can manage your stress and control your diet at home to alleviate IBS symptoms.